CANCER SURVIVOR
WARRIOR QUEEN

Marilyn S. Floyd

Edited by: Sarah Germain Lilly

authorHOUSE·

AuthorHouse™
1663 Liberty Drive
Bloomington, IN 47403
www.authorhouse.com
Phone: 833-262-8899

Published by AuthorHouse 07/12/2021

ISBN: 978-1-4567-2050-6 (sc)
ISBN: 978-1-4567-2049-0 (e)

Library of Congress Control Number: 2011903008

Print information available on the last page.

I want to dedicate this book to my children:

JULISSA: JULISSA's sister, who died, was born in the same month on the same day as Julissa. She is a gift to me from God, an angel born again.

Chante: Chante is a talented child. She has many gifts, not just from her mother, but from her father. Her father was a "jack of all trades, master of none."

Denzel: I know Denzel is going to be a business owner. He always talks about buying me a house one day. I can't wait.

Devonte: I see Devonte as a professional architect designing and building buildings.

Donavin: I see Donavin as a judge helping lots of people all over the world.

Daven: I see Daven becoming a business owner. Daven cannot take orders from anyone.

FOREWORD
THE WARRIOR QUEEN

My name is Warrior Queen. I am a three time cancer survivor. The first cancer I had was nasopharyngeal that was in the back of my nose. I received chemotherapy and radiation. I was only eighteen years old at the time.

The symptom I had before I knew I had cancer was swollen glands. I went to the doctor and was given medication to ease the swelling. Two weeks passed and the swelling did not cease. I began developing pain in my head. It was so painful that I could not sleep at night. My mother took me to a specialist. The specialist sent me to get a test in which the results showed that I had cancer in the back of my nose. I felt as though my life was over. I did not cry because I was unaware of how serious it was.

> My mom and aunt were really calm. They would talk with each other privately because they did not want me to know exactly what was happening. Before leaving the doctor's office, I was given a date to return to the office to begin my first chemotherapy treatment/session.

When we got to the hospital I had to change into my nightgown, then the nurse came in to start an IV before my chemotherapy. I was really nervous, but I knew I had to get myself together. I did not know what to expect. All I remember was when the medication entered my body I grew more anxious, then I felt nothing. Within the first thirty minutes I began to feel nauseous and spitting up all over the place. My nausea would increase when I smelled food. I was given medication to help with the nausea. That was not a good feeling.

A week later, I was combing my hair in the bathroom and as the comb ran through my hair once a large amount of hair fell out. I ran the comb through my hair once more and more of my hair began to fall out. I broke down crying, but I managed to pull myself together and decided to just comb all my hair out. I was bald and all the hair on my body had fallen off. My mother had a wig ready for me because she already knew my hair was going to fall out. The wig was just right for me. I loved it. The wig was long, curly and black. You couldn't tell me anything. It made me feel a lot better.

A week after that, it was my last week of chemotherapy. I did two weeks of chemotherapy. I went home to get ready for my radiation therapy. I started that Monday morning. I started getting nervous all over again. My mother, my aunt and I arrived at the doctor's office and the nurse told me to remove my clothing, again. I went into this room that had all kinds of big machines. As I wondered what's next, the doctor came in and told me to get on the table and put my hand in a big, round machine. I was very scared at first.

The doctor marked my face with a magic marker in the areas that the treatment would be given so that every time I received my treatment the area was already marked. I had to wear the magic marker on my face when I went outside. I felt really bad all over again. People would stare at me everywhere I went. I would always try to hide my face and sometimes I would just cry. Some people were not nice at all. I had to wear the marker on my face for six weeks straight. Family, friends and strangers looked at me funny. That was not a good feeling at all, especially because I am used to looking my best. Then I finished my six weeks of radiation therapy.

Then over the years my teeth started decaying one by one. Eventually I had to take out all my teeth due to radiation therapy. I started feeling really bad again, walking around with no teeth before I got dentures. Having no teeth in your mouth as a young girl like me with a nice shape, good looking and a pretty smile. My teeth were perfect. I could've starred in a toothpaste commercial.

Not only all my teeth came out, but I also lost some hearing in my ears as well. I have to wear hearing aids in both ears. People will talk to me and I cannot hear their words clearly. Before I knew I had hearing problems, I had to look at their mouths and listen very carefully. I felt really sad and on top of that I had speech problems as well. When I talk a lot of my words are not clear. Sometimes my speech improves when I eat food. It helps my words sound clear. Since I know that eating food helps me talk better, I make sure to eat food to clear my throat before speaking with someone.

Having speech problems, people that do not know me hear me talk and look at me like I'm dumb. They look at each other like "what the hell did she say?" or they laugh at you with each other. Specifically, when you are with your guy friend the girls are the worst. Girls always find something on you to make you feel bad. It made me feel so bad I would cry when I was alone. I would even stay home and refuse to go out if it was not to the doctor's office. Having a speech problem made me depressed and not want to be around other people.

If only you knew. It's a hurting feeling. People who have a disability should not be looked down on and judged because it is unknown how that person's disability developed. I think people should be more compassionate and mindful of how they treat people like me and other people with disabilities. It can one day be them. We are no different than anyone else. Please do not look down on me. I can be your mother, sister, aunt or friend. I love you. Do you love me? I'm thinking. I went through the first cancer having teeth removed, speech problems and then skin problems from the radiation.

The radiation burned the head and neck area of my skin. It even damaged the tissue, leaving blood clots and nerve damage. My skin is hard to heal due to damaged tissue from the radiation therapy. This is another problem I am dealing with. I wear turtlenecks or scarves to cover my neck. I cannot wear sexy dresses with neck openings like other women. Being young and seeing other young girls wearing those beautiful dresses that I wish I could wear made me so sad. I even went to some specialists for skin. They really didn't want to give me plastic surgery. Every specialist I went to said I am high risk and should not have plastic surgery. I decided to listen to their recommendations and I left it alone. I was living day by day with my skin looking like I was in a fire.

Just when I began to think my problems were over, I got cancer again in 2016 in my neck area. They had to remove my thyroids on my right side, leaving me with more damage to my neck. Knowing I had cancer again, all kinds of thoughts were running in my head. I was thinking about my children and grandchildren. I was scared, worried and indecisive about what I was going to do. I had a lump in my neck that had to be removed. The doctor told me the outcome of the biopsy. That made me so scared again. I was thinking about if I'm going to make it and worrying about who's going to care for my children if something happens to me. That is not a good feeling. No parent wants to think about that.

I said to myself if I don't have the surgery within a certain time frame, the cancer can get even worse. I did not want it to worsen and I began to think about how many people depend on me such as my children, grandchildren, friends, family and people I may not even know. I started praying and asking God to guide me in the right direction and give me the strength to go through the surgery without harm. God answered my prayers and gave me the strength to go through the surgery without harm. I came out with a great report. There was one percent chance of developing cancer again in my thyroid. Thank You Jesus.

I began thinking that everything is alright again. However, I had to get a second surgery because I developed a bad infection in my neck area. I was in the shower when I saw something that looked like inflammation and I did not know where it was coming from. When I got out of the shower, I saw yellow pus running down my neck. I was so scared. The first thing I did was call my doctor. They told me to come into urgent care as soon as possible. When I got there, the nurse instructed me to put on a hospital gown. Afterward, the doctor came to tell me what he was going to do next. I was very nervous like always. Then I went back into the surgery room. They had to scrape me out.

After the surgery, I had to spend a week in the hospital. When I was discharged, I had to have a nurse come to my house to take care of my open wound until the wound closed. Then, I started to feel better. It's always something. I'm thinking everything is okay again. I am cancer free. I was mistaken yet again.

Ding dong. Hello. I'm colon cancer. Don't forget about me.

What do you want again? I started having stomach pain, constipation and blood in my stool. Every time I used the bathroom the blood in my stool increased. My doctor scheduled me to get a biopsy. The results came back positive. I was very very sad again.

When it rains it pours. The doctor told me they were going to put a plan together for me. I had to have two procedures performed on me on the same day. I was so so scared again. Another major surgery. I went home. The nurse called me back in to talk with the surgeon. The surgeon team mapped out where they were going to do the surgery, where they were going to scrape out the cancer cells and take a biopsy at the same time. The surgeon then asked me what day I wanted to have the surgery on. I had planned February. I was trying to take as much time as possible. I really didn't want another surgery. I thought about my children, family and friends that needed me. I play a big part in people's life. They really depend on me.

The number one person I look to for everything is God. God is my rock. Without him, I would not exist. God gave me a life to live. A life to make a change in my children's lives and others. So, I ask God for the strength to go through surgery once again. I had my surgery and came out of it like the warrior queen I am. Glory be to God. Amen. Thank You Jesus. You are my rock.

After my surgery was over I had to be scheduled for chemotherapy. I started my chemotherapy on February 17th. I haven't had chemotherapy since back in the 1980s. I didn't know what to expect for the treatment because of the new technology. I went in for my treatment and the nurse called me to tell me everything she was going to do. I was very nervous at first. The nurse started an IV in my arm. It was very difficult to find a vein in my arm. They had to get a good vein so the chemotherapy can go right through. If the chemo is not going in the vein it can burn your arm and cause extreme pain. The nurse finally found a good vein after sticking me three to four times. I was so happy the nurse found a good vein. I was already nervous about if it was not the right vein. I did not want to feel any type of pain.

First, the nurse put a bag of liquid steroid fluid to help with the nausea I may feel from the chemo. Then, she started the chemo fluid and it moved slowly through my veins. I laid back to relax, although I was still nervous. I didn't know what I was going to feel. The nurse put warm bags on my arm to help. She made me feel very comfortable and it helped ease my anxiety from the beginning to the end. The nurse was great.

After my treatment was over, I sat down for a while to see if I had any side effects. The only thing was a little nausea. My pressure was very high and I felt weak. My daughter Chante Fulmore was with me every step of the way during my chemotherapy. She is my caretaker as well. I was rolled down in a wheelchair because I was weak. A cab came to pick us up. My daughter, granddaughter and I got in the cab.

We were riding for a bit and got a few blocks from the hospital, when suddenly a big sanitation truck hit the cab on the side I sat on. I just finished my chemotherapy not feeling good at all and then got into a car accident. That was the worst day ever. I had to go back to the hospital. I was in so much pain. The car accident made me sick. I got home in the morning. My daughter and granddaughter had to go to the emergency room. I will never forget that day.

The next day, I had to start my chemotherapy pills as well. The pills were medium sized pills. I had to take four pills in the morning. That was four thousand milligrams. Then I had to take four thousand milligrams at night after dinner. I already hate taking pills. I had to take the pills for three months, twice a day.

Now, I have to deal with COVID-19. When it rains it pours. I still had to go to get my liquid chemotherapy every two weeks. I'm taking two kids of chemotherapy. I was so scared because so many people were dying like flies. I felt like giving up. It was like everything was falling apart. I was scared that I would get the virus. They were saying people who were getting chemotherapy, diagnosed people with heart problems, and elderly people can contract the virus. I did not want to go outside at all.

I talked with my doctors and nurses. They assured me that I was going to be safe coming to the hospital. I got the courage to go outside to receive my treatment. I was almost finished with the treatment. All I thought about was my children. My family and friends need me to be there for them.

I had to start praying more to God to keep my family, friends and I safely through this crisis. I want to thank God for giving me the courage and strength to go through my trials and tribulations. It has been a long one. The battle is not mine, it is the Lord's. God has a plan for me to touch and to be an inspiration to family, friends and others.

CHAPTER 1

WARRIOR QUEEN

I love my self, ever since birth I been trying to find myself. It seems like I am caught up in this crazy world. Somebody help me please. Is it something I am doing wrong? Is it because I am too black or too white, happy, sad, or too nice? I am studying myself like "What is the purpose I am on this earth? I know it is for a reason." I went to just about every church just trying to find who I am. Going through so many things in my life, I know I am not doing it by myself. There is a higher power. I look back as I write this book. It helps me face a lot of things I been going through in my life. I did not know how bad the problems I was in were. It takes one strong woman or man to overcome or deal with their problems.

Today I have no teeth, lockjaw, stiff neck, poor circulation, speech problems and hearing problems. Sometimes we ask our selves why do things happen to me?

I don't have food, I have no car, I don't have those sneakers, I don't have a house.

You have to be thankful for what you have. Somebody is always doing worse than you. Somebody is bed bound, somebody doesn't have legs, an arm, eyesight is gone. Somebody got nowhere to stay, got no food, homeless. You have to thank God for what you have.

When I was a little girl growing up I dreamed of being a model or professional dancer. Another thing I like to do is help people with any problem that they might need help with; in my kid's school I just help the principle out, teachers, anything I can do in the school. My son asked me am I going to move with him when he goes to college? I said "yes"; I was just joking. I have six beautiful children. I thank God for them, I can't ask for anything else. I am blessed.com. You have to stay busy doing something to keep your mind active and have faith in God. You can forgive but you can never forget. Stay the same person. Never let nobody change who you really are. Live your dreams; life is what you make it.

I hope you enjoy the story of my life.

CHAPTER 2

EYE TO EYE WITH THE DEVIL

Have you ever heard a ghost story about someone seeing something that seems unreal to the human mind? Well, it happened to me in real life. When I was five years old, I had a life experience that I would never forget.

It was 1972, and I lived on Throop Avenue in Brooklyn, New York, with my cousins Andrew, Mark, Joanna, and Daisy. Well, I didn't live there—it was just that I was always over there. My aunt Doris didn't mind me coming over. Her family was very close to me. My cousins were like my brothers and sisters.

It was one very hot summer night on East New York Avenue. My cousins and I were all playing around. Joanna and Mark were doing scary pranks. "Muffy, go into my room and pull out the talking doll," Tommy said and laughed. "Muffy" was my nickname, which people called me because of my puffy cheeks. I got the name from my grandmother.

Joanna teased me. "She's not brave enough to do it."

I stared into the room. It was so dark. I decided not to go in there. A little while later, we all went in together. I saw a glow on the left-hand side of the room.

I ran full speed and dived under the covers. I poked my head out. Andrew, Mark, Joanna, and Daisy were standing and staring as if they were watching a horror movie. I was hoping this wasn't one of their pranks, because the shivers were running down my spine.

A chilling sound struck my ears. It was a rattling sound. I held my blanket as tightly in my fists as possible. A rattlesnake sizzled out of the

3

wall. It was bursting full of colors, like a cartoon. The snake suddenly began to transform. It became three beautiful horses. They were as white as snow and had wings like an angel. They were like horse-men, part human and part horse. They had human faces, but the rest of the body was that of a horse. One horse had a black man's face; the other horse had an Indian's face, and the third a white man's face. I started to loosen my grip on the blanket. It seemed like they were harmless.

I wondered, *Is this real? Can they harm me?* All these questions were spinning around in my head. The horses started to join together and became a small red head. As the white horses got closer to each other, the head kept swelling until it resembled what we would call the "devil."

The head was so red! I gazed over to see if I was the only witness. My cousins' mouths were wide open. The sight of the creature's face was too much to handle. My hands shook faster than my heart was beating.

The head had horns that were as sharp as knives. The man's eyes stuck out, and there was flaming hot fire in them. There was a beard on the tip of his chin that came to a point at the end. This thing, whatever it was, looked like it hated the world, or at least us. It was so supernatural!

The head looked directly at us and said, "Boo!"

My uncle Arthur came into the room with the dog when he heard us yelling and screaming. The monster was gone. I couldn't sleep the rest of the night thinking about the devil coming back. We all squeezed into one bed.

The next day, we talked and talked about what we had seen. My hands were still trembling from my encounter with that face. The face looked like a ball of hate and evil. I couldn't take my mind off it. None of us could. Where was God when this happened?

Little did I know I would see this devil along the way in my life in different forms. I learned to let go of the covers I held to my cheek no matter what. I learned that the monster can't hurt me because of the God in me.

CHAPTER 3

ROBBERY

It was 1974, and I was seven years old. I was finally living with my mother and my brothers and sisters. My mother, Joseph, Andrea, Stuff, Muller, and I were living on DeKalb Ave in an apartment building. Next door to our house, there were dope addicts.

One sunny morning, my mother left us in the house to go to work. After my mother had been gone twenty minutes, there were two knocks on our front door. Joseph and I went over to the door and asked, "Who is it?"

No one responded. So Joseph turned to leave. Before he took another step, someone knocked on the door twice more. "Who is it?" I asked.

"Umm, your mother sent me for the television," a man said.

We didn't open the door. One of the men pushed in the door. There were two guys with knives in their hands. My own hands started to shake. I was so terrified. I didn't know what they were going to do with us.

One of the men grabbed each of us by our arms one at a time as hard as he could. He forced us into the closet. All of us stood in the closet waiting for someone to rescue us. I kept crying and crying. I'd never experienced anything like it.

We heard a bed being moved toward the closet. These guys were pushing it to the closet to keep us in. I peeked through the little cracks in the closet door. I saw them snatch the television cord out of the wall and carry the TV out the door. The guys struggled down the hall with the television.

When they finally left, we were wondering if we should come out of

5

the closet or wait. We were all so scared. It took about five minutes for all of us to make our way out of the closet. That afternoon, when my mother came home from work, she lay on the couch and kicked off her shoes.

"Hay, Mom! We were robbed by those dope guys from next door!" I yelled as quickly as possible.

"They told us to get in a closet, and they had a knife!" Stuff blurted out.

"Ma, they stole our television!" I complained.

After everything was explained, my mother called up her brothers: Michael, Buck, and Peewee.

When they finally got over to our house, we explained what had happened again. My uncles came up with a couple of friends and went searching for those guys. They first checked next door to see if they were in the pool hall. Then they went around the block. They walked down the block as if they were gangsters or famous hood cats. Peewee finally spotted one of the guys. There he stood, joking around with three of his friends.

"Hey, fellas! I think one of you guys has a TV that doesn't belong to ya'll," Buck said.

"Uh, what you talking about, man?" one of the guys said.

One of the men looked nervous and guilty. Michael reached into the side of his pants. They must have thought he was about to pull out a gun, but they were wrong.

Michael pulled out a long stick and ran toward the dope heads. All eight men ran after my uncles. My other two uncles followed behind Michael. Even though my uncles went down there, it didn't change the fact that we didn't have a television.

They must have sold the television for some dope. Anyway, the week after that, we all moved from DeKalb Ave. What surprised me was that the building was burned down right after that and many families died. Thank God we moved, because if we had stayed, we could have been among the victims to die in the fire as well.

Every day, I think about how blessed we are to be alive. That's how I knew that my family was blessed—not only because we were spared from the fire, but also because when the robbers came into our home, they could have raped or killed us. But thanks to the grace and mercy of God, that didn't happen.

I could not sleep for days, always thinking someone was coming into the house while we were sleeping. I felt so scared. I would be looking for someone to come through the window, just seeing the dope bandits nodding like they were going to fall down. I thought I had to catch them before they fall—that was even more scary.

CHAPTER 4

FOSTER CARE

The year before in 1973, we were living on Elgin Street. One day, my mother started arguing with the Puerto-Rican lady upstairs because of her two sons. The lady didn't believe what her sons had done to me.

My mother was ready to beat her butt, because her sons had tied me up with handcuffs trying to touch my body. They had tricked me to go and play with them in their apartment. Good thing my cousin was looking in the peephole in the apartment. My cousin went to get my mother. My mother ran as quick as she could to get me out of that apartment.

The lady ran full speed down the stairs calling the cops, because my mother had taken the garbage can and set it on fire. She was trying to make the lady come outside.

Five minutes later, the police and fire department were racing down Elgin Street.

"You stupid-a-- b---!" my mother exploded into words. "No one told your stupid a-- to call the cops. They can't stop me, dumb b---!"

The cops got out of their cars and observed what was happening.

"Lady, I am going to have to tell you to move away from the fire," one cop said.

My mother did as she was told. The Puerto-Rican lady went running down the street shouting, "This crazy b--- tried to kill me and my family! She set the garbage can on fire and planned on throwing it at me. I didn't want violence from the start, but she won't stop." She shivered.

"Oh hell no! I did not do sh-- to that bimbo!"

"Who da hell you calling a bimbo, ho?"

My mother was trying to explain herself, but the police didn't want to hear her. When they got there, they saw she was trying to set the garbage on fire.

The police demanded they stop talking and arrested my mother. I stood by my window while the police were putting the handcuffs on her. I instantly ran downstairs crying.

"Why are you taking my momma? Oh please don't take my momma!"

My mom was just trying to stop the two boys from touching me on my body parts.

"Your mother will be fine. Tell your brothers and sisters that you guys are going to camp for a while."

I knew that we weren't going to camp and so did they. We were going to a group home for kids with no parents.

When we got to the foster home, there were so many rules. One of them was no wetting the bed. We all knew this was going to be difficult for Muller and me.

When the lady left, I whispered in Muller's ear, "Do not wet that bed. Make sure you use the bathroom before you sleep. I love you. Good night."

I lay my head on the pillow and cried silently. I just wished that my mother was there with us. I started dozing off to sleep and began to dream.

"Splash!" went a loud sound. It was my pee hitting the floor!

That sound woke me. Then I heard Muller getting beaten. The lady swiftly came to my side and dragged me off the bed. She whipped me until tears scattered on my cheeks. My heart was beating fast. Then Stuff spotted Muller and me getting whipped with a belt.

"Hey, you can't do that!" Stuff yelled.

"Well, I can do whatever I want as long as I am taking care of you dirty kids."

"You are not my mother, you old bat! Let go of them!" Stuff said.

Stuff got a spanking after arguing with the lady, but it was not as bad as what Muller and I got. We had whip marks all over our legs.

That afternoon, we heard that our grandma was coming. Muller and I wore long pants to cover up the scars.

"Grandma! Oh, Grandma!" we cried.

"Hey, babies, I'm going to take you guys home with me soon, don't worry." My mother was there too! I was so relieved to hear those words out of Grandma's mouth. We all smiled and looked at each other. All types of questions were roaming through my mind. But first, I had to blabber about how that crazy old lady had almost beaten us to death.

Then Muller told my grandmother and mother what the lady been doing to us. My mother burst out again "Where is that b---? I am going to kick her --ss." The supervisor came into the room, and my mother charged out of the room trying to get the lady. The police came again. I knew they were going to take my mother again. The case worker took the lady out of the back door. I never had been so happy in my whole life, They gave us to my grandmother. We didn't go back, and the lady could not get any more foster kids at all.

We finally arrived at the police station to give a statement. My mom was all shackled up. She didn't look as good as she usually looked. The policeman escorted her to the room we were in.

"Hey, honey, how you holding tight?" Grandma asked.

"Mom, don't worry about me. Please take care of my babies for me. I don't want them in that home with people they don't even know. Oh please, Ma," Mom begged on her knees.

I couldn't believe I was seeing my own mother begging for help. This was a side of my mother I had never seen.

"Look, child, you got yourself in this, and now you got to get yourself out. Now, I will take your kids for the benefit of them."

"Thank you, Mom. I promise I will get myself together."

Being in a foster home, I don't wish that on nobody no time. It's not always the best place to be. I want to say to anyone who has to go into a foster home if you are being abused always let someone know. It can't get no worse than it already is.

"Now, kids come over here, give your mother some love," Grandma said.

Muller, Stuff, and I ran to her, wrapped our long arms around her, and held on tightly until we were weak.

CHAPTER 5

FRIENDS/ENEMIES

The move to Classon Ave in Bushwick was a lot. A popular Funk musician used to be in the basement of the building I used to live in, and my aunt Pauline and David used to sing with them. As soon as I moved back to St. John St. when I went outside one evening, the kids teased me. I wore dirty clothes, and my hair was a mess.

I was upset that we had moved back to St. John St. in Bushwick. My mother couldn't buy all six of us clothes to wear and I had to do my own hair. My mother was always hanging out on the street. One day, as I was playing outside by myself, a girl came across the street. She looked like she was getting everything she wanted. Her hair was straight, and her clothes were nice and clean.

"Hey, how are you?" the girl said. "I see you're playing by yourself. Can I play with you?"

"Umm, sure, okay," I mumbled.

"My name is Melissa."

"Oh, my name is Muffy." I smiled.

Melissa's mother then came outside and told Melissa to come inside to eat. Her mom then said that I could come too. After we ate, Melissa's mother wanted something from the store and I said that I would go for her. I came back from the store and Melissa's mother gave me money for going to the store for her. Boy, that was all she wrote. I started coming over to Melissa's house. Melissa to clean her room, and I used to volunteer to clean Melissa's room for her. I knew Melissa's mother was going to give me money. I didn't do it just for that, I did it because I was feeling good that I could help Melissa out. Her mother was giving me her old clothes and shoes. I remember the time me and Melissa were playing outside with the other girls and boys. We were playing tag. One boy was chasing me, and then he picked me up, trying to carry me up the stairs at another friend's house. That is when I fell out of the boy arms and hit my head on the concrete ground. Blood started leaking down my face, and I ran to Melissa's house, screaming. I thought I was dying. I was so scared that I didn't know what to do.

Melissa's mother took care of me. I didn't need stitches, but it left me with a bald spot in the front of my head. I have to cover my forehead with my hair, so you won't see the spot.

Months later, Melissa and I became best friends. She and her family were the only people on the block who respected me as a person. Melissa's sisters, Pauline and Jewel, was treated me like a little sister. It was like I was a part of their family. I slept many nights with Melissa and her family house. Melissa paid for me to go to the movies with her.

One day, as Melissa and I started playing tag, some girl came across the street.

"Hey, Lissa, how come I haven't been seeing you lately?"

"What's up, Denise? This is my friend Muffy." Lisa beamed at her.

Denise gave me a stink look.

"I'm your best friend, and best friends don't leave each other," Denise nagged.

"Look, I'm the only friend she has, so be a little considerate please."

Denise looked familiar. *Oh my gosh,* I thought, *she one of the girls that teased me on the block.* She was with this other girl who had thrown dirt into my hair and teased me about by clothes. I didn't say anything, because I didn't want her bothering me again. Denise did not know that Melissa had told me about a girl Denise who's mother was a call girl. "That means she slept around for money" Melissa told me. No wonder Denise had so much jewelry and so many nice clothes all the time! They were not legal residents of the United States.

Melissa invited me to her house again.

"You are so close to me, Lissa."

"Yeah, I know. You're like my sister." Melissa smiled widely.

Her smile was as wide as the Kool-Aid smile. I loved her so much. Her family treated me as if I was a part of the family. They treated me better than my other people that lived on the block. As we grew older, Lisa and I grew apart. I met new people, and she did as well. Michelle and I became the best of friends too.

CHAPTER 6

When I was just a teenager I met this man named Vincent. Vincent was much older than me; he lived by himself. Vincent worked at a warehouse in Queens, he use to make shoes. Vincent brought me new shoes home every day. He used to buy me everything I wanted. I think I was the only young girl in the area who had dated a older man. I was so embarrassed when I was with Vincent because he was so ugly looking. At least I thought so, but he had a nice personality. My brothers use to tease me about him, even my mother said things about him.

My mother even tried to hook him up with my aunt Della. Vincent didn't wanted nobody but me, he told my mother. Vincent had friends named Elijah and Danielle. We used to do everything together, Danielle and I. We would go shopping and get our hair done. We also went out to parties together.

Elijah and Danielle used to sleep over at Vincent's house a lot. One day, Elijah came over when Vincent was not home. I was there by myself. Elijah came knocking on the door. I asked who it was.

He said, "Me."

I asked, "Elijah, what do you want?" He said he wanted to ask me something. I opened the door, and then I said, "What?"

Elijah said that he liked me and wanted to be with me. I was so surprised. I'm thinking to myself if they wanted a four some. I was not having that at all.

When Vincent came home, I told him right away. Vincent was already a jealous man. His friendship with Elijah fell apart. Vincent didn't want Elijah over to the house anymore.

Vincent and I never told Danielle. Elijah and Vincent met each other on the outside of Elijah's house. Me and Danielle's friendship fell apart so fast. I was close to mother and father too. They were wondering what happened to our friendship. We still did not say anything to anybody. I felt so bad because I used to love Danielle and Elijah like brother and sister.

One day, an old girlfriend of Vincent's named Eve came by the house looking for Vincent. The bell rang and I went to the window. I asked who it was. No answer. I asked again, and then Eve spoke up. I asked her what she wanted. Vincent came to the window asking her what she wanted. She wanted some money for her birthday. I told Vincent not to give her anything. Then she said "I am not talking to you."

Then she offered me to come down the stairs, talking about how she is going to beat my butt. I went down the stairs, and she came up to me and put her hand all in my face. I had no choice but to punch her in the face.

My mother said "Never let them get the first punch." I always remember that. I told her to pieces. Then I just beat her butt up.

Then the next day, her cousin came to my house with ten to twenty girls saying that I was talking about her. I then said, "If I have anything to say to you, I'll say it in your face. I am not scared of you either."

Then, one of the girls, Coney, tried to put her hand in my face. I started swinging, hitting anybody and everybody who came my way. Then two weeks after that, Coney came back again talking about her man.

Was I talking to her man? she asked. I told that girl to get the hell out my face. Then she put her hand in my face, and I had to beat her butt again. After that, Coney never bothered me again.

I met another girl by Vincent's house. Her name was Marcher. I used to hang out with this Marcher girl too. We went to the park to play handball together. I used to give her clothes and help her out with food she did not have. Marcher would ask me to do her hair.

After all we had been through, this b--- turned around and slept with Vincent. I found out because Marcher did tell me a guy gave her gonorrhea, That is how I knew she slept with Vincent. He had given it to me too. I was so f-ing mad if I had seen that girl, Marcher, I would have broken her ass up into pieces. That girl hid from me for weeks and months.

I did not want anything to do with Vincent anymore. I was leaving Vincent's home when he ran in back of me; then he jumped in front of me saying that I was not going anywhere. I pushed him out of my way.

He went into another room. I did not know what he was going for. The next minute's Vincent came up to me with a gun. He hit me on the head with the gun and said, "You are not going to leave me." Boy, I have never been so scared in my life.

I went back into the house. I was only being nice to him that night because I knew the next day I was going to be gone. Oscar went to work that morning, and I got the hell out of there. I went back home with my sister and brother. Vincent came home from work looking for me, but my ass was gone.

I did not see Vincent for weeks. I knew he would come looking for me. I had used my head. I went to meet another man a lot bigger than Vincent. Vincent came by my house on Rector Street; that was when my mother was staying there. I was with my other friend in the room having sex with him. I did not know that Vincent was there knocking on my door. My mother did not know that I had Stanley in my room. My mother opened the door to let Vincent in.

Vincent came to my room and knocked on door. I was butt naked. He saw that Stanley and I did not have any clothes on. Then Vincent left the house. I was so happy to get rid of him. They won't mess with another man.

My mother liked Vincent very much because he used to buy my mother's love. Back then, my mother loved some money. Vincent never came back to my house again.

I want to let young and older women if you scared of a man that is violent meet another man that is much bigger than him. It worked for me.

CHAPTER 7

ALFRED

I was dating this guy named Alfred. He was very nice at first—or I thought he was. Alfred showered me with gifts. He bought me everything I wanted. He was a very strange man. I liked him very much until he followed me into the bar across from where I lived on Rector Street. It was a place where transit workers used to hang out. The transit workers all knew me and my family; we all were like family.

Alfred used to wake my mother up at night crying and saying that I was cheating on him, which was not true at all. I had not given Alfred a reason to be jealous. One day, I walked across the street to the bar to make a phone call. I did not know Alfred had followed me into the bar. He was right behind me. As soon as I stepped into the bar, my sister friend Tyron said, "Hi," to me.

That was when I heard Alfred in back of me saying, "Ooh, that what you be doing in here? Talking to men?"

I said, "You do not know what you are talking about.

That is it. I am finished with you."

Alfred started walking behind me crying and crying. I walked back across the street, but *Alfred made it back before me*. Joy's father drove up in a car. He had come to see Joy. I went to the car and said, "What's up, Roy?"

Joy came over and talked to her dad for a while. As soon as Roy left, Alfred smacked the shit out of me. That was all he wrote. I jumped all over him and started beating his ass up in the street and back into my hallway. That was the end. I could not have taken it anymore.

I told Alfred I was not going to see him anymore. He left and then came back over to my house saying that he was sorry. He asked if I could come to his house to do his laundry for the last time. I said I would do his laundry for the last time not knowing Alfred was setting me up all that time. I went downstairs to the basement where Alfred's room was. He was waiting in his room for me. He opened the door and said, "Come in."

I went in. I asked Alfred where the clothes he wanted me to wash were.

Then Alfred grabbed at my hand. He then start saying "Ooh my god, why you going to do that to me? I love you. Please don't leave me." He started to pull down my pants. He said, "Oh my god," and asked me why I was talking to that guy. He was bugging out. He kept trying to take my pants down. I finally got Alfred off me somehow. He picked up a hammer and tried to hit me with it. I ran into the bathroom as fast as I could and pushed the door closed. The door did not have a lock on it. I was holding it with my feet. Alfred was kicking the door trying to get in.

I had never been so scared in my whole life. I finally said, "Miss this. I have to get out of here somehow." I kept saying to myself, "Run as fast as you can up the stairs." I just opened the door and started running. I kept running until I reached all the way outside. Then I ran so fast home, just crying. I was so scared. I told my mother, and she called her mother, my grandmother, who sent over my uncles Michael and Buck and their friends. They went to Alfred's room looking for him. Alfred was not there, but his friend, who had been there all that time and did not help me, was. My uncles and their friends trashed Alfred's room and friend.

The next day, Alfred had a pastor from a church call me. He said that Alfred was sorry about what he had done. I told the pastor to tell Alfred not to bother me anymore. Alfred promised he would not call me anymore. That was the end of that.

CHAPTER 8

RECTOR ST

When I was living on Rector Street, my sister's boy friend's friend liked me, but I didn't like him. He was from Jamaica.

I came into the house, and he said, "What's up, girl?"

I said, "Nothing."

He tried to play with me. I told him to leave me alone. He kept playing with me. He was not listening to me, and I got mad. He saw that and said, "Move ya blood clot." He still wasn't listening to me. He put his hand on my face. That was all he had to do; the next minute, I picked up an antique glass thing and busted it in his face. I got so mad I didn't know what I was doing. He was bleeding. There was blood running down his face.

My brother and sister tried to break up the fight. I cut my sister's finger with a glass pitcher by mistake; that is how mad I was. He was still trying to fight me, but he couldn't. He was fighting like a little punk. I thought I was going to jail. The next day, he told me if it hadn't been for my sister's baby's father, he would have shot me. I told him to go somewhere. "You ain't doing nothing." Back in the day, I was no joke. I didn't take shit from anybody. I was living on Rector Street in Bed-Stuy.

My mother left me and my sisters and brothers by ourselves to live with a man named Traver. We were so scared. We didn't really know what was going on. My big sister Andrea had to go down to the welfare office to have the rent check come in her name.

Because Andrea was the oldest girl, she was like a mother to us. She

23

made sure the house was clean, the laundry was done, and food was on the table.

Andrea and I didn't get along at times. She used to curse me out. I felt Andrea was being too hard on us. She used to make us clean. She did not want us to go outside. Andrea wanted everything done her way. I didn't have any clothes. I was wearing the same clothes every day; she wouldn't get me anything new. She would let them treat me like anything. Tony had a friend who would come by, and one day, he was sleeping in my bed at the bottom. I went to sleep on the same bed.

I think he had sex with me while I was asleep. I never told anyone. I confronted him, and he ran out of the house. That was the end of that. One day, I was sitting outside. It was summertime, and an old friend was driving by. We were pretty good friends, or so I thought. He took me to his building on Sutter. It was an apartment building. He told me to go with him into this building. I thought we were going to the movies.

I went into the building with him and up to the second floor. He opened this door, and there were naked women and men in the room. I acted like I had not seen this. I told him I had left something in the car. I went downstairs so fast. I walked all the way home. I did not have any money or a phone on me. It was dark outside, and the building looked like it was abandoned. It was another lesson for me.

Before that time I lived on Lawrence Street, I met this girl. Her name was Ann.

We would play handball in the park across the street from where we lived. At the time, handball was my favorite sport. I was very good at it. I played every day. Ann used to smoke reefer. She asked me to try it. I took two puffs and got so dizzy I could not stand up. I kept falling down. The room was spinning around. I felt like I was going to die. Even when I lay down, the room still sp. Finally, I went to sleep. When I woke up, I felt much better.

I had tried reefer before, and it never made me feel like that. I think somebody put something in that reefer. Ann left me in her house alone. For all I know, she could have had me raped or something; I was that out of it. I don't know what happened after that. From that day, I never smoked reefer again.

I used to like this guy named Ricky. He was a DJ. Ricky was light-skinned and sexy. He was also very popular.

One day, I went up the hill on Marion Street where Ricky was saying. Ann went with me that day. There were so many people there you couldn't move; that was how crowded it was. Ricky came to me to ask me to meet him at his apartment. I was waiting there. It was right where he was staying.

Ricky then came and took me upstairs. He told me to wait in his room. I was waiting. He went out of his room for minute. I started hearing noises, like someone was yelling. That was when I found out Ricky had a girlfriend.

I heard her saying, "I saw you with that b---. Where she at?"

Boy, I was scared. I ran out of the room when they went outside. Ricky took her up the block somewhere. All I know is I ran down the street as fast as I could. The next minute, I heard gunshots. I started running even faster. I had never been so scared in my life. It felt like I was running for dear life. I didn't want to see Ricky anymore. I was so happy to get rid of that problem.

I also met a girl named Renay while I was living on Lawrence Street. We were the best of friends. Renay and I used to hang out.

We would go up the hill where the guys were hanging out. There was this one guy named Supreme. Boy, he was so good-looking. I had a crush on him. Supreme and I started getting close. One day, Supreme asked me to come to his house. I went. So we were chilling and watching TV. Then we started kissing. I didn't know how to kiss at the time. He tried to take my pants off. I didn't know what to do.

He asked me, "Are you a virgin?"

I told him, "Yes."

Then he pulled down his pants and to tried to put his dick in me. He couldn't put it in. After a while, he started moving his ass, and I guess he came. I got up. I was bleeding, and I was scared. I didn't know what had happened. I thought I was in love after that. I was so embarrassed.

My mother met this man named Ale. She met him driving down Bushwick. He was riding a truck looking for scrap metal. He was a nice guy.

He put a baseball team together. My mother and all of her sisters—Doris, Candy, Della, Deborah, Janice, Tee bone, and Karen Green—played, and my sisters and I were cheerleaders. The team name was the Laws of Nature. Boy, we had so much fun. My mother's team used to win a lot of games. One team my mother's team used to play got mad at my mother; they even wanted to fight her and her sisters. There were too many of us, included my uncles and cousins. I loved cheerleading. I was in charge.

I never had so much fun in my life. Watching my mother play baseball, I felt so happy. I cheered when my mother hit the ball. She could run fast too. We used to practice every day, and people looked at us. Our uniforms were yellow and green. We went home with trophies. After a time, my mother and Ale broke up; that was when the baseball team went down and everybody started doing their own thing.

When I used to live on Rector Street, I went to JHS 277. My sister Andrea used to go too. Andrea stayed in trouble. She cut classes and did not go to school. When I first got into 277, my grades were A's and B's; after a while, I started following Andrea, cutting class and not going to school, just hanging around.

There was this one girl named Lynette. She was a big troublemaker. Lynette was also a bully. I was not scared of anybody, because my sister and friends were in the same school. Lynette was picking on a girl in school, and I told her to leave her alone. Lynette told me to mind my own business. She got in my face; that was all she wrote. I grabbed her and started kicking her ass. From that day, Lynette didn't bother anybody in the school. I used to help people who were getting bullied.

Lynette and I became friends. I don't hold anything on people. I always try to keep the peace. There was another girl who said something to me in the school. She was a Puerto Rican. I didn't do anything to her in school, because I knew I would get in trouble and I didn't want that. I told her to wait till after school. I told my friends what had happened.

They came to the school and beat the girl up badly. They cut her up. I didn't tell them to fight her. They were supposed to come up there in case someone jumped in while I was fighting. I came out of school and did not see the girl. Somehow, they found the girl that day. I was scared to go up to the school. I thought I was going to get locked up. The teacher did not know I was involved in the incident.

I never saw the girl again. I think her family took her out of school. Ever since I started fighting in school, I never took any mess from anyone.

All the guys used to try to talk to me. I was popular. I made a name for myself. There was this girl who lived across the street named Melody. She and I became pretty good friends. Melody lived with her mother and brother and sisters. There was a bar downstairs from Melody's. We knew everybody in there. There were several transit workers in there. I used to go make phone calls in there. They had a pay phone.

CHAPTER 9

ONE-WOMAN JOURNEY

In 1981, I was seventeen years old and dating a Jamaican guy, who was much older than I was. He had dated a lot of other woman before we met. I was very fond of him, and I grew to like him a lot. James was in love with me. He was so in love with me that he gave up all his other women to be with me. His mother preferred one of his other girlfriends to me, since she was financially more independent than I was. She hated the idea that her son had chosen me.

All the times I visited James's home, he never introduced me to his mother. I felt very uncomfortable being in her house and not having met her, so one day, I asked him why he had never introduced me. He told me that he would let me meet her someday and not to worry about his mom. I kept seeing him.

One day, I went to James house to do the laundry. I walked out into the hallway, and it was dark. James' mother, Ms. Brown, ran toward me and threatened me.

"If you come back in my house, I'm going to do you something." I was young and told myself that she was not really going to kick my ass.

I told James about it, but he told me not to worry about his mother. He said that he paid his mother's rent, so she couldn't tell me not to come back to their house. I listened to James.

Weeks and months passed quietly. I kept going to James' house, and soon, James' mother became friendly with me. We started doing each other's hair, and I bought her a gift on her birthday. I loved her. She used to make me these special turkey dinners all the time. I enjoyed it very much, but soon after one of these turkey dinners I got a terrible pain in my right ear.

I went to the doctor, and I was diagnosed with an ear infection. It kept getting worse so I went to see an ear, nose, and throat specialist. The doctor said he had never seen anything like it before. He said there was a growth in the back of my nose. Since it was in the back of my nose near my skull, surgery was not an option. After the diagnosis, James' mother told me to go home to my mother to let her take care of me.

I was admitted to the hospital and underwent months of radiation therapy. James never visited me. His mother visited once. Two years later, after I had recovered, Mrs. Brown came to visit me at my house. I was happy to see her after such a long time. She brought me strawberries and other fruits. I introduced her to my three-month-old daughter, and her father, who was my boyfriend at the time. During Mrs. Brown's visit, my boyfriend and I went out to pick some things up at the fruit stand. We left Mrs. Brown to visit with my sister, Andrea, and Joy.

I told them that we'd be right back and asked Stephanie to give Joy her bottle if she woke up. Later, Andrea told me that Mrs. Brown took Joy away from her, did not give her the bottle, and instead, rocked and mumbled to Joy. When we got back from the fruit stand, my sister and I started talking about Joy's christening and which one of us would buy the dress. Mrs. Brown offered to buy the christening gown, and I told her yes. The christening was set for February 7.

Two days before the baby's christening, on February 5, I called Mrs. Brown to ask her if she had gotten the christening gown yet. She told me that she still had to hem the gown. I thought that it seemed a little strange, but Mrs. Brown brought the gown the next day. Joy was christened on February 7 as planned. On February 8, I found the baby suffocated. She looked swollen, and she had unusual marks on her face that reminded me of the character in the movie *The Exorcist*.

After Joy was buried, her paternal grandparents, my aunt, and my mother were talking and wondered if maybe Mrs. Brown had done something to the baby's gown. After all, Joy had been a healthy baby. The paternal grandparents were Jamaicans, and they took the christening gown to a reader/advisor. She told them that Mrs. Brown had done something to the gown and that it needed to be destroyed immediately. Weeks after the funeral, I contacted Mrs. Brown and told her that Joy had died. She acted as though she did not care, in contrast to her behavior when she had visited just before Joy died.

I realize now that Mrs. Brown had never accepted me in her family at all. She had been putting on an act all those years. When I think back to when I would stay with James at their house, I remember feeling like she was always watching me. I remember hearing creaks at night in the floorboards of the room next to James', which was not her bedroom. Every time I tell the story, I scare myself. I think of all the time I lived with her, and she was feeding me those special homemade turkey dinners.

The cancer treatment I went through left me with scars all over my neck and into my chest and shoulders. I can't hear out of my right ear, and the hearing is going in my left one. I have lockjaw now, and I am embarrassed to go out and eat in front of other people because I can't open my mouth very wide. My voice has changed, and it is difficult for me to speak clearly enough to teach my children. She could not kill me, so she tried to harm my firstborn daughter, Joy, who was born November 25, 1987.

After Joy died, the relationship between her father and me died too. On November 25, 1988, God blessed me with another daughter. I named her Joy. After going through a few bad relationships, I found out that life isn't bad after all, and I am still the same strong woman I always was. I met a man named Ty, who showered me with wonderful thoughts. He was and is down-to-earth. He is the type of guy who opens the door for me, and his heart is like a flower.

I know that where there is a strong man, there is a strong woman, but through all my experiences, I learned that you must never give your soul to anyone. The devil is always waiting to collect your soul, but he is never going to collect mine. I am just hanging on for dear life.

CHAPTER 10
MARRIED TO FRANK

I used to work as a home attendant helping elderly people. Once day I got off work heading home. I had to take the bus to get home. Across the street from the bus stop was a driving school. I just got my permit. I said to myself, I need to start taking lessons to learn how to drive. I walked across the street. I went inside the driving school. Inside it has all prices for driving lessons and 5-hour class. I was just looking around to see how many lessons I might need to take. That is when Frank came out and said "May I help you with anything?". Then I said "I just got my permit, I need some driving lessons. I was just looking over your prices. I do not know how many lessons I might need." Then Frank said "let me take you for one driving lesson and then we go from there." Then I said I would come back when I am ready. I left my phone number and I took one of Frank's business cards. I went back across the street by the bus stop. I had to run because my bus was coming.

When I got home my daughter Joy was waiting for me. I was a single mom. I had to work to make sure I could provide for her. Her father Sam and I had broken up because of his jealousy. I was on the phone with a friend but he thought it was another man. It was not. When I saw that, mind you, I was with a guy before him and the man was very jealous; I know the sign of being too jealous and it can lead to stress or somebody getting hurt. That is why I ended it with Joy's father. I was not dealing with no jealous man at all. If you can't trust me, we can't be together. That is another story… Couple of days went by then Frank called me and asked me when I am going out for a driving lesson. I then said I was still not ready. Frank said "Okay, let me talk you out for one free driving lesson." I thought about it. I said "A free lesson, okay, I can go out this Saturday at 1pm." Then Frank said "I will see you on Saturday."

Before Saturday came, Frank called my phone and asked me to come downstairs. I said "Okay give me a minute." I got dressed and then headed down the stairs. Here Frank was in the front, sitting in a nice car. He was dressed nice and smelled so good. I was impressed with Frank. Then Frank asked me to dinner. I was like 'hell yes!' to myself. Then I said yes. Frank took me out to a nice place. The food was so good. Then Frank took me home. Then from there we kept dating going out to different places.

Then I started going out for driving lessons. Frank was a good teacher he took his time with me. Days went by and my driving was improving very fast. After my driving lessons, I had to do the 5-hour calls. Then Frank scheduled me for the road test. Before the road test Frank had to brush me up. I took the road test and passed the first time. I was so happy after I got my license you could not tell me nothing.

Get out of the way people there is a new driver on the road!

Me and Frank continued to date. I started going to his office and helping him out. Frank treated my daughter Joy as if she was his own. We started going out like a family. Frank did so much forJoy and me. I met his brother and kids. We started going down south every summer to visit his mother. His family felt a way about me because I was much younger than he was. Frank was 20 years older than I was. They probably thought I loved Frank because he had money.

Time went on and Frank asked me to move in with him. So I did, with my daughter Joy. His place was very messy. I finally got the apartment together. I cooked, cleaned and went to work with Frank. He told me to stop working. I didn't stop at first but then I did.

One day I found out I was pregnant by Frank. I was in my first stage of the pregnancy. I didn't want another kid at the time because I wanted to wait until I was married. I didn't tell Frank I was pregnant. I got an abortion. Then days and weeks went by and I got pregnant again. Then I told him what I did and told him I didn't want any more kids until I got married. Weeks went by and I was helping Frank out in the office. He came in there with his best friend Kingsley and gave me a ring then said "Let's go get married." He had all the papers ready to go. We went to get married, then we went back to work as if it was a regular day.

Time went on I gave birth to my daughter Chase, then I had a son then years after another son. Then the next year I gave birth to twin boys. Boy I thought I was running a nursing home for babies. I had to shut the kitchen down. No more babies. My husband bought me a big house in a nice area. He opened up a new driving school and insurance company not far from the house. I went to school to get my insurance license and Frank opened up a driving school in my name. I was working in the office and we had the kids in the office as well. I had a bed for the kids to lay down in if they got tired. I stayed home with the kids more than I stayed in the office. The kids were a lot of work.

Frank ran everything in the office. Later on Frank bought another house. Frank put it in my name. Time went by and Frank decided to put the house in his name. I didn't understand that. I told Frank "No you have one house in your name. I am going to keep this house in my name." Then I started to look at Frank different. It was like he thought I was dumb because I was much younger than him. Like he thought I didn't know better. When I told him I was not taking the house out of my name all hell broke loose. We started having problems. Frank was coming home late. Things were not feeling right anymore. Frank was trying to run everything down to the business trying to keep me home all the time. I noticed I would go by the house because we had three tenants living in the house to get the rent money. They said they did not want to give me the money. They would only give it to the owner, which was my husband Frank. I left from the house and waited for Franks to come home from the office. When he got home I asked him why he told the tenants not to pay me rent. I said to Frank I am the owner of the building. Then he said nothing. Days and months went by, me and Frank was on bad times.

He was not helping me with the house. I still will go over there trying to get the money but the tenants was still not paying for me. One tenant had her daughter throwing garbage outside and papers out the windows. I was getting tickets after tickets from the Sanitation Department. To make a long story short then we went to Landlord and Tenant court. I was trying to get them all out so I could sell the building. I thought, if I sold it me and Frank's relationship would get back on good terms.

I was wrong. I sold the house and things got worse. Frank did not come home. I was up all night waiting for him. Something told me to go by his friend mother's house. I knew he went over there to drop off money for his son but I would always think Frank was seeing her. Time to find out; I got in my car. I called my sister and told her to meet me over there. I just knew Frank was over there. I headed to Frank's baby motherhouse. When I got there any my sister was not there yet so I drove around to see if could find his car.

I spotted his car, then started calling Frank's phone. He still was not answering. Mind you, I had my son with me. I took him out of the car and then put my son in the stroller headed to the building where Frank was at. I remembered the floor she lived on so I waited for someone to come out to get in. Finally, someone came out and I headed to the elevator. I found out it was broken and I had to walk up the stairs to the top where Frank was at then started heading to the door that I thought was Frank's baby mother door. No answer, so I started banging harder and harder. Nobody opened up the door. So I headed back down the stairs, tired like hell. As soon as I got down the stairs my sister was there waiting for me. Then Frank came from the door exit. He saw me and headed to me. I'm asking Frank, "What the hell you doing here?"

I said to Frank, "I should cut your ass up." My sister said "Don't do it!" Then I headed home. I thought Frank in the kid's room. I had nothing to say to him at the time. I then noticed the house locks looked loose, like someone was messing with the locks. I started fixing the locks. The more I fixed them, the more they became loose. Then another day the window was wide open. When I went to check the door I closed it. Another day my son kept crying and crying. I knew he was not going to stop until he got his bottle. I was headed down the stairs when I looked straight ahead by the window in the den. When I saw someone opening them up. So I yelled "Get my gun!". When I started yelling I turned the light on and I called the police; I was so scared out of my mind. My husband never came down or anything. Then the cops came.

CHAPTER 11

FROM BAD TO WORSE

I told the cops what I saw at my window. Then the cops asked if me and my husband were having problems or if I have any enemies. I said me and my husband was having problems. I know I did not have any enemies at all. I treat everyone very nice all the time. All the time the cops where there my husband stayed upstairs. The cops said they would hang around for a while. I said okay. I was still shaking. I stayed up all night; I could not sleep. Sometimes I would stay up until I see the light. Then I would go to sleep. I did that for a couple days. I then notice in my daughter's room, the door going out to the porch had the lock broken. I was scared again. I asked Frank if he can fix the lock; he did nothing. Mind you, I am up all night until I see the light. Frank never put the lock back on the door so I asked a neighbor. The neighbor said he would come by to put the lock on but he never came.

For that night I got a stick and a leather belt. I tied the belt on Joy's bed and to the door just like a rope. The next day I woke up went to Joy room and the sliding door was open half way. I asked Joy if any of them opened it. She said no. Then she said she heard a noise and was scared so she went back to sleep. Hearing that made me more scared.

Days and months went by and I went back to work. I stared going in the office more regular. It was Joy's graduation the week coming up. I had to go buy a dress and shoes. Then I had to get her hair done for prom. We started getting dressed all up so nice. Joy looked so pretty with her pink dress, black shoes and her pretty hairstyle. We were about to leave out only one thing, we left the camera by the office. We had to go get the camera at the office. We pulled up in front of the office.

Frank got out first. Then I jumped out because I had to use the bathroom. Frank put the key in the door. I was in back of Frank. Next minute I felt someone behind us push Frank and me into the office, reading Frank his rights. I was so scared. I did not know what was going on. The officer put Frank in one room. Then another officer took me to the lobby of the office. He started asking me what I was doing with an ugly mother-fucker like Frank. I was surprised to hear that coming from an officer. I just looked like "okay." The officer said he was going to check to see if I did not have any warrants. Twenty minutes went by the officer said they were letting me go. They opened the door and let me out. I went as fast as I could to the limo where the kids were. I had to drive the long limo home. We owned the limo. We got out the limo went in the house. The kids did not know what was going on. Joy missed her prom day and I felt bad for her. I did not know what to do because I had never experienced this before.

I called his oldest son and told him what happened. Then I just waited there for Frank. I found out a couple days later that Frank was doing a lot of fraud on taxes, selling no good insurance and fake licenses. I could have gone to jail because I had my insurance license and driving school license as well. They had been watching Frank. I said what else do I not know about Frank? When you think you know a person. Frank was still in jail. His friend came by to drop off some mail that came from Frank's old office. Then I said "Let me look inside the bag." When I looked inside, it was mail for me from the tax people. I opened the envelope. I knew I never filed taxes before because Frank said I never made enough to file. I read the letter.

It was asking for more info from me for them to send the money to me. Mind you then, I was searching for my business name on paper. I didn't see it. Frank used a company name that was out of business. Boy, I was so mad. Again, we were still on bad terms. I said to myself "This is it. We done." Frank finally got out of jail. When he came home I asked him "Did you file taxes in my name?" He looked around as if he did not know what I was talking about. Then I showed him the mail. He looked surprised and asked me where I got it. I said the bag of mail that your friend dropped off from your old office. Frank looked at me dumb and said to me "Yes I did it. If I would have asked you would've let me do it." Then I said "You have no right to invade my privacy." I wanted to knock Frank out. I threw Frank out the house. Then it was hell to pay.

Frank was so mad, hell, I was so mad. Frank started having people mess with my alarm at the office. Mind you, I threw Frank out the house and the office too. I kept going to the office every night to turn off the alarm and then a couple days later Frank came by the house. He was saying it was his house and he wanted me out. I said I was not going anywhere. Then Frank started cursing me out like a dog. I went back in the house. Mind you, Frank had people coming in the house when I was not home through the window. The bathroom window would be open and the lock tampered with. I was scared. My mother had lived in the basement at the time and my mother had to move out because I think Frank flooded the basement by busting the pipes. My mother lost a lot of her furniture and clothes. I stayed at the house just me and my kids, no one to defend us but God. Amen. I was doing work in the house, and things were all over the place. I was making changes in the house.

My husband then had the lights turned off in the house because the light was in his name. I went down there to try to put it in my name but it took days before it could happen. The light was still off but they was going to come. The same day ACS worker came out. When it rains, it pours. When the lady came to my apartment it was upside down. Frank knew I was working on the house. He had someone put in the lobby a dead mouse and dirt. The house really looked bad. I did not leave it like that. It was upside down but not like that. I showed the ACS workers what Frank was doing but she told me she was going to take the kids if I knew what Frank was doing. She said it was like neglect. She then said she could send someone to pick us up so I could get away from him.

Then I said okay. She told me she would send someone in two days. I did not want my kids to be taken from me so I got together a couple of things in the house. I left really everything behind. I was tired of everything Frank was putting us though. They put us in a domestic violence shelter. We stayed there for 6 months until we got an apartment. Being in a shelter for the very first time was scary. I did not know what to expect. Our whole life had changed from there. I no longer worked for myself anymore. I was no longer a homeowner. When we first got into the shelter, they had rules we had to follow. No visitors at all. You had to be in for a certain time. You have to meet all the staff members. Inside the shelter, they gave use clothes food and we met different people like other families who were in the shelter. We had our own apartment room. They came around every morning to inspect the room to make sure you were keeping the place clean, had no drugs and to make sure everyone was in their room

There were people in there not following the rules at all. They were not coming in on time, and having drugs in the shelter. Some were being put out with their kids and it was so sad to see. My kids at the time had to go into a new school and they met new friends. I had started a new job working on a school bus, but I had to quit to take care of my kids. It was not easy. I hung in there until I was accepted to section 8 and then I had to look for an apartment. It was very nice. It was not so bad being in a shelter at all, what you put in is what you are going to get out. I know there always two sides to a story.

CHAPTER 12

HARASSMENT

One day, I went to the emergency room at Long Island College Hospital, located at 339 Hicks Street in Brooklyn. There was a man in the emergency room who was a transporter; he was observing me from near the door.

He had come to my bed to ask me if everything was okay.

I told him, "Yes."

My sister Tony was with me at the time. He came back over a second time to ask me personal questions about my life. He asked me if I had a boyfriend. I gave him a look because I felt he was getting too personal. Then he made a comment on my eyes. He said, "You have some pretty eyes."

At the time, I didn't pick up the hint that he was coming on to me. He left and returned to say that he was going to transport me to my room. Once he had taken me upstairs to my room and I got settled in, he said he would come back and check on me.

Before he left, he patted my hair down and looked at my sister to tell her I was beautiful. That was when he left and repeated he would be back to check on me.

Twenty minutes after my sister Tony had left the hospital, he returned to the room. While in the room, he pulled a chair up to my bed.

He then asked me what was wrong with me.

Then I told him my neck was swollen, and he said, "No, your leg is swollen," and put his hand under my cover to rub my thigh. I was puzzled at the moment.

I was saying in my head, *This guy is not being friendly. He is just trying to come on to me.*

I told him not to rub my leg.

Then he tried to kiss me twice. That was when I told him to leave and not to return. There was another patient in the room with me. She thought I knew this person. I told her I did not. Then she told me to call the head nurse to file a complaint, which I did. Then the head nurse came to my room. I explained to her what had happened. she said she was going to get back in touch with me.

I called my sister Tony to explain to her what had happened. A half an hour later, Tony and my nephew Lorenzo came back up to the hospital, which I didn't know. She was talking to the head nurse to explain what she had seen. She was very upset that had happened to me, knowing how sick and weak I was.

As Tony was talking to the head nurse, she saw the man who had harassed me. My nephew Lorenzo was getting ready to go punch him in the nose. The guy looked at Tony and then stormed out of the emergency room.

He didn't know my sister was in the room, and he came right back to my room and asked me what had happened. I explained, "You weren't trying to be helpful or nice. You know what you did." He tried to say I accused him of that because he was white.

He said, "Oh, because I'm white."

And I told him it was not because he was white.

As I was telling him to leave again, the head nurse walked in and warned him not to come to my room for anything. He did not want to leave my room; the head nurse had to call security. After they escorted him from the building, officers from the Seventy-Sixth Precinct came by to take a report.

When I was released from Long Island College Hospital, I went to do a follow-up with the officers in the Seventy- Sixth Precinct to see what had happened. They said they would get in touch with me. No arrest was made. I felt like I had been discriminated against because I was a black woman making a complaint. I felt like the officers did not do their job. That man was free to keep on being helpful to other female patients.

I had to get help. I needed a home attendant to help me and my children after my second minor stroke. The social worker told me that the ACS had to be involved, because I had children. The caseworker came out first; the visiting nurse came out after to help me start the paperwork. Later on, the ACS worker came out. First, it was a lady. I had her for one month. Then they changed my caseworker. I don't know why. They gave me a man's name: Elias. He was very nice at first. I thought he was being too nice. Elias was coming by too much. I started getting mad. I thought he was being nosy. I felt he was coming by if I was doing something with the kids. I noticed Elias would hug me every time he came by. Every week, he would come by. I found that to be strange. I found out he was coming by because he liked me. The last time he came by, he brought the kids something from the center sneakers and pajamas. He said they were giving t hem out at the center. Before he left my house, he hugged me again and then gave me his house number so I could call him. I called him only one time. The next week, he called me asking if I would be in the area, as he was going to pass by. I told him that I was in the area, and I would be home soon. I pulled up at my house, and Tobias pulled up at the same time. We all got out of the car and went up the stairs. Soon, we entered the apartment, and Elias gave me another hug. The kids went into the room to do their homework. Elias then said to me that he could not have a relationship with me, but if he had met me before he had my case, he would have had something with me. I said it was fine with me because I was not feeling him anyway. He was basically trying to cover himself, because he went back to the agent saying that I was coming on to him. I did not know he had done that until another ACS worker, a lady, replaced him. I asked her what had happened to Elias. She asked me right away if she could go to the bathroom. I showed her where the bathroom was She then came out of the bathroom saying, "Can I talk to you for a minute?"

I took her to my room. She asked me if Elias and I had had an argument.

I said, "No."

She asked, "Did you all get along?"

I said, "Yes, we got along."

Then she said that he had told them that I was trying to come on to him. I could not believe it at first. I was so surprised he would make up something like that even though he was coming on to me. I told the lady what had really happened, about him coming on to me. It was the other way around. I hit the roof. I even got sick be hind that. The caseworker then told me to talk to her supervisor. I did, and she told me to come file a report. I went down there the next day with my cousin Rommel. He must have done it to someone else too. I went down there to do a follow-up; the caseworker said he no longer worked with them. Then I left. The whole thing was he thought I was going to tell on him about him coming on to me.

CHAPTER 13

LORENZO

On September 16, 2007, about 3:15 a.m., a detective called me to tell me to go to my sister's house because my sister was very upset.

I asked them, "For what?"

That was when they told me my nephew had been killed. I remember it was like someone had killed one of my sons. The police didn't know that Lorenzo was like my son too. It was like the whole world had left me. I dropped the phone. I started to panic, screaming and yelling, looking for an answer. Who did it? I even lost my teeth that day. (I wear dentures.)

Even to this day, I never found my teeth. I stayed without teeth for two months. I was not worried about any teeth anyway. I still do not believe my nephew is gone. I had one minor stroke after that. I was deeply depressed.

People would ask me to go out, and I would make excuses not to go out. I didn't know I was depressed until I asked myself, "Why am I not going out?"

That was when I found out that I was in a depressed mode. I wasn't facing the fact that my nephew was gone. I tried not to think about it. I hurt so very much. I had to pull myself together for my children. Lorenzo was like a big, brother some kid, especially to Joy. They were not just cousins but best friends too. Lorenzo made sure we were okay. He even treated me like I was his mother

He would never disrespect me for anything in the world. I felt like I had let Lorenzo down, because I didn't want him to move in with me. . Lorenzo knew that I was always strict with my children. Still, I would have given him anything he wanted because he loved and respected me.

"I miss you so much, Lorenzo. Rest in peace, Lorenzo ..."

CHAPTER 14

A TIME FOR SHARING—WARRIOR QUEEN

It was back April 8 1982. that was the day that I was diagnosed with nasopharyngeal cancer. I was only **eighteen** years old at the time and very frightened to hear this diagnosis. My treatment consisted of two weeks of chemotherapy, followed by seven weeks of radiation. It was a difficult time in my young life. Like most people undergoing treatment for cancer, I suffered from side effects. First, I needed to have teeth removed, and then as a result of the radiation, I suffered from blood clots and damaged tissue in my head and neck areas. I also lost some hearing, and to this day, I have difficulty moving my head from side to side. I also continue to have speech problems.

However, one of the most frightening things was when the doctor told me that I might never be able to have children. Fortunately, he was most definitely wrong. On November 25, 1987, I gave birth to a baby daughter. Sadly, Julissa died the day after her Christening on February 8, 1988. The doctors said she died as a result of crib death. But through God's benevolent grace and mercy, I was blessed with another daughter, who was born on the exact same day and month as little Julissa. And as time went on, I was blessed with five more children, including a set of twins.

After a marriage of eleven years filled with mental and physical abuse, I was forced to leave my home and live in a shelter. I was a victim of domestic violence. I went from being a homeowner of ten years to being homeless. Together, my husband and I had owned a small insurance company and a driving school. However, my husband was an unscrupulous man, and eventually, we lost everything. I'm presently on disability raising six children on my own. It's not easy, but I am doing it.

My children are my inspiration, and they keep me strong. Each of these experiences—the cancer, the loss of my first daughter, my stay in the domestic violence shelter, the sexual harassment, and the broken marriage—both the trials and the triumphs, have contributed to helping me become a stronger person. To anyone who has cancer or any other problems, it is so important to tap into your inner spirit, the source of life that can only come from God. Yes, you have cancer, but try to adopt an attitude of gratitude for what you have and use the resources around you to encourage and inspire you. If you believe in God, *stop*, *think*, and realize that God has a plan and purpose for you.

Live to love, not to complain or worry or to be angry or in denial. Embrace the challenges that confront you, and use them to propel you into learning how to experience the lessons of living in the moment. The physician and medical team members can administer medical treatments to you, but how you respond mentally, emotionally, and psychologically depends on *you*! Think positively, and help others. Count your blessings to help relieve your stress and depression.

Make a decision today not to dwell on the unfortunate things in life but to go forward and soar into new beginnings. Because it begins with one positive thought: I *will survive*! No matter what happens, I know that with God's help, all things are possible because I believe! I want to leave you with this message regardless of your circumstances: there is always hope. Never give up.

www.ingramcontent.com/pod-product-compliance
Lightning Source LLC
Chambersburg PA
CBHW020407290526
45785CB00005B/2462